Helichrysum Essential Oil

Benefits, Properties, Applications, Studies & Recipes

by Ann Sullivan

Published in USA by:

Ann Sullivan
217 N. Seacrest Blvd #9
Boynton Beach
FL 33425

© Copyright 2015

ISBN-13: 978-1545130148
ISBN-10: 1545130140

TABLE OF CONTENTS

Introduction 9

Chapter 1: Benefits of Helichrysum Essential Oil 15

Cultivation of Helichrysum 15

A History of Helichrysum 16

Chemical Components..17

Main Properties of Helichrysum Essential Oil........18

Antioxidant...18

Antiseptic..19

Anticoagulant...19

Anti-inflammatory...20

Antibacterial...20

Antifungal...20

Antiviral 21

Antispasmodic 21

Anti-allergenic..21

Anti-catarrhal 22

Astringent...22

Nervine 22

Diuretic 23

Expectorant...23

Mucolytic 23

Cicatrisant...23

Hepatic...24

Common Therapeutic Uses 24

Detoxifying Agent.....................................24

Skin Care...25

Respiratory Issues....................................25

Cardiovascular Wellness............................26

Digestion 26

Relieving Allergies 26

Safety Precautions & Common Applications..........27

Safety..27

Blends...28

Chapter 2: Recipes for Helichrysum Essential Oil.....29

Pure Applications 30

Abscess Tooth 30

Agitation 30

Aneurysm 30

Anxiety..30

Bleeding 31

Bone Bruising or Pain...............................31

Broken Blood Vessel 31

Bruising...31

Catarrh 32

Cholesterol Levels 32

Colitis 32

Cramps...32

Cuts 33

Depression 33

Detox 33

Earache 33

Gallbladder Infection...33

Hematoma..34

Hemorrhaging..34

Herpes Simplex..34

Hernia 34

Hopelessness...35

Joint Pain 35

Ligament Pain or Injury 35

Liver Support...35

Lymphatic System Cleanse 35

Heavy Metal Detox 36

Muscle Aches 36

Nosebleed...36

Pain...36

Pancreas Support..37

Perseverance...37

Phlebitis 37

Psoriasis 37

Scar Tissue..38

Sciatica 38

Shock/Trauma....................................38

Sinus Infection....................................38

Skin (Dry, Sensitive, Eczema, Fibroids,
Dermatitis, etc) 39

Staph Infection 39

Strength 39

Stress 39

Stroke 40

Swollen Eyes 40

Tendonitis...40

Tennis Elbow......................................40

Tinnitus...41

Tissue Pain & Repair 41

Varicose Veins 41

Vertigo 41

Viral Infections...................................42

Wounds...42

Blends 43

Arthritic Massage Oil 43

Brain Stimulant...44

Facial Salve...45

Gum Inflammation...46

Headaches 47

Hemorrhoids 48

Hot Flashes...49

Muscle Ache & Pain..50

Pain Relief..51

Pregnancy & Delivery 52

Seasonal Allergy Blend......................................53

Scar Salve 54

Scar Salve II 55

Stretch Mark Salve 56

Sunscreen 57

Sunscreen II 58

Tennis Elbow 59

Varicose Veins...60

Wound Healing 61

Chapter 3: Helichrysum Essential Oil Studies 63

Study 1 – Antioxidant Properties 64

Study 2 – Anticancer Properties 65

Study 3 – Fatigue/Burnout 66

Study 4 – Antimicrobial Properties.............................67

Study 5 – Antifungal Activity 69

Study 6 – Insecticidal Properties 71

Chapter 4: The Ins & Outs of Essential Oils 73

Where do essential oils come from? 73

How are essential oils extracted? 74

   Pressing Method 74

   Distillation Method 74

   Solvent Method 75

   Maceration Method 75

How do you use essential oils? 75

   Topical Administration 76

   Inhalation Therapy 77

   Ingestion 78

What are the general benefits of using essential oils?
....78

   Replacement for Prescription Drugs 78

   Cost Effective Supplement 79

   No Expiration Date 79

   Versatility 79

Conclusion 81

Introduction

What are essential oils, and how might they be used for therapeutic purposes?

First things first, essential oils are natural and organic. They are derived from the significant compounds found in the plants that possess them. Seeds, bark, flower petals, stems and roots, as well as other functional parts of the plant, can all be used to extract essential oils from a given plant. All of us have experienced the aromatic properties of the plants that provide essential oils, even if we are completely unaware of what was taking place when it happened. Remember the last time you bought, or received, a dozen roses? That beautiful aroma exploding from the roses, is just a part of the aromatic properties and qualities of the essential oils that can be extracted from that particular flower. In conjunction with providing specific smells to certain plant species, essential oils also offer plants a layer of protection against diseases and possible predators. They also have a significant role to perform in the pollination procedures of the associated plant species.

Essential oils are not water based. They are actually phytochemicals consisting of the powerful fragrant compounds of the plant. Phytochemicals are the compounds that occur naturally within the plant itself. This means that there are no synthetic additives, which are common in conventional medicines. Essential oils are fat soluble; however, they do not possess the same fatty acids or lipids associated with animal or vegetable oil products. Essential oils are extremely clean, pure products that absorb into the skin almost immediately upon being touched. Essential oils are translucent when unadulterated and have a color range that spans from crystal clear to a deep and vibrant blue hue.

Here is an experiment you can try at home. Take a fresh lemon and slice it in half. Peel the rind from the fruit and squeeze it between your hands. That aromatic fruity smelling residue left behind is chock full of ingredients used to make essential oils.

Essential oils should not be confused with fragrance producing oils or perfumes. Essential oils are natural and organic and are taken directly from the plant. Perfumes and fragrance oils are either artificially created, or manufactured with synthetic solutions and do not possess the same therapeutic properties as essential oils. Essential oils are super concentrated substances, which means that a very little, usually a drop or two, will go a long way. The aromas and chemical compounds associated with essential oils allow them to provide therapeutic benefits for both physical and psychological procedures.

Essential oils are offered by a number of manufacturers and distributors around the world. They vary in price and quality, which is determined by a number of different factors. The country of origin for the plant species being used, how rare the botanical is, how much oil can be produced by a specific plant, growing climate present for the plants, and standards applied by the distiller/manufacturer, will all play a very important role in determining price and effectiveness of the essential oils being produced.

Essential oils are generally sold in small bottles or vials separately, or in slightly larger containers consisting of essential oil blends. The benefit of buying blends is that you can eliminate the need to purchase all essential oils separately. The disadvantage of buying blends is that you have no control of the mixture.

Chapter 3 will further detail past scientific research on helichrysum essential oil.

Now, let's get down to it.

Essential Oil 101: the Basics of Helichrysum

Summary: Helichrysum, or Helichrysum italicum, has been traditionally used as a detoxifying agent, because of its anticoagulant and anti-catarrhal properties. The oil can help detox the liver, lymph, gallbladder, and blood. It also helps with circulation of blood and regeneration of skin, making it an ideal support for skin issues, bruising or swelling.

Description: Helichrysum oil is commonly extracted through steam distillation. The flowers are most often used. The oil is light yellow in color, thin in consistency, and has a somewhat strong fresh earthy scent.

Uses: Beyond those applications previously mentioned, additional uses for helichrysum essential oil include supporting the body's natural defenses against acne, burns, dermatitis, wounds, abscesses, boils, cuts, eczema, and other skin irritations. It also helps support the body's defenses against atherosclerosis, blood clots, arteriosclerosis, hypertension, phlebitis, muscle pain, hematoma, hearing, cholesterol regulation, liver disorders, bladder infection and muscle and bone inflammation. When it comes to mood and emotion, the scent of helichrysum promotes security and peace of mind.

Properties: Antioxidant, antiseptic, anticoagulant, anti-inflammatory, antibacterial, antifungal, antiviral, antispasmodic, anti-allergenic, anti-catarrhal, astringent, nervine, diuretic, expectorant, mucolytic, cicatrisant, and hepatic properties.

Application: Use neat or undiluted. You can apply topically, inhale directly, diffuse or use as a dietary supplement.

Safety Precautions: Helichrysum has been approved by the FDA for internal consumption and so can be used as a dietary supplement. However, if pregnant, do not use this oil.

Fun facts: Helichrysum is derived from the Greek words for "to turn around" and for "gold," which are "helisso" and "chryros." The flowers were so valued that the Greeks would offer helichrysum flowers to their gods.

And the flower is valued for more than its essential oils today; the shape, color and fragrance of the helichrysum keeps so well when dried that the flower is often used in displays.

Chapter 1:
Benefits of Helichrysum
Essential Oil

Helichrysum essential oil offers a number of therapeutic benefits; but you may be wondering what these benefits are. In this chapter, we'll take a closer look at the history of helichrysum and its many uses.

Cultivation of Helichrysum

Around 600 species belong to the genus, Helichrysum, which is a member of the sunflower family, Asteraceae. Many of the species occur in Africa, particularly South Africa, along with Europe, Asia and Australia. Helichrysum italicum is the species from which essential oil is often extracted. This perennial flowering plant comes from the daisy family and produces an aroma akin to curry, due to the pungent scent of its leaves. Growing in the Mediterranean, helichrysum thrives in rocky or sandy dry soil. The plant can grow up to 60 cm tall, but most are low-growing yellow-flowering clusters, which are used as much for aesthetic purposes as for practical ones, such as for dried flower arrangements, due to the fact that they keep their color long after they're picked.

A History of Helichrysum

The name, "helichrysum," is derived from the Greek words "helisso" and "chrysos," which mean "to turn around" and "gold," respectively. This plant is sometimes used as a spice. Although the plant smells like curry powder and is therefore called the "curry plant," it is not used in curry or masala dishes and has no relation with the curry tree, which is not even of the same genus (Murraya koenigii). Instead, the bitter aroma is perhaps more akin to that of sage, which also more closely directs its similar uses as a seasoning. The leaves and shoots of the plant are used in various types of Mediterranean dishes – vegetable, meat, or fish. They are often stewed so that the dishes might absorb the flavor, and then pulled out prior to serving.

Although historical applications and records about helichrysum are few and far between, there are some culturally and therapeutically significant facts worth mentioning. In Italy, helichrysum is used to flavor sauces and is said to produce a combination of a curry, alongside a slightly delicate rosemary tasted.

In South Africa, helichrysums have long been used in traditional medicine to support inflammatory issues, like rheumatism. The Afrikaans believed that the flowers lasted for seven years, thus naming the plant the "sewejaartjie" – "sewe" meaning seven and "jaar" meaning years. The names "Everlasting" and "Immortelle" are also common terms for this plant, due to its ability to retain its yellow coloring.

The plants have also served as digestive fuel when mountain climbing or as potpourri for their distinctive scent.

Helichrysum blossoms produce an oil that is used in essential oil, fragrances, and perfumes, but the history of helichrysum when it comes to uses in essential oil is even scantier than its general historical records, because helichrysum only became an active oil in the aromatherapy industry during the early 1980's. The oil has become a popular one in present-day use, however, with more and more research being done on helichrysum to identify its uses and understand the mechanisms of its efficacy.

Chemical Components

In order to generate the essential oil from helichrysum, the flowers must be steam distilled. This results in the oil's key chemical components, which are primarily linalool, d-limonene, a-pinene, b-pinene, geraniol, nerol, furfurol, g-curcumene, b-carophyllene, neryl acetate, geranyl acetate, eugenol, isovaleric, italidone, and diones.

Main Properties of Helichrysum Essential Oil

Along with the properties previously mentioned in the introduction, helichrysum oil possesses antioxidant, antiseptic, anticoagulant, anti-inflammatory, antibacterial, antifungal, antiviral, antispasmodic, anti-allergenic, anti-catarrhal, astringent, nervine, diuretic, expectorant, mucolytic, cicatrisant, and hepatic properties. With such a versatile range, helichrysum is well equipped to fight off any pathogen in the body's path.

Helichrysum, as mentioned, is composed of linalool, d-limonene, a-pinene, b-pinene, geraniol, nerol, furfurol, g-curcumene, b-carophyllene, neryl acetate, geranyl acetate, eugenol, isovaleric, italidone, and diones. These components are what instill the enormously beneficial properties within helichrysum essential oil. We'll outline these properties below.

Antioxidant

Anything high in antioxidants – whether fruit, beans, or essential oils – is a powerful advocate for your body. Antioxidants both protect against free radicals and repair their damage. What are free radicals? Free radicals are destructive chemicals that invade your body, produced by substances both inside and out. Some free radicals (or oxidants) form through normal bodily reactions, like inflammation, metabolism and aerobic respiration. Other free radicals form outside the body, but enter it due to exposure. These include harmful pollutants, toxins, smoking, alcohol, X-rays, and UV rays, to name a few. Although our bodies produce their own antioxidants, these often become damaged as we grow older; thus, introducing antioxidants into our bodies allows these nutrients and enzymes to assist in chemical reactions which destroy the oxidants or free radicals. Helichrysum essential oil is a moderate antioxidant, aiming to detox the body of free radicals that lead to disease. Click here to read a study on the oil's antioxidant properties.

Antiseptic

The antiseptic properties of helichrysum essential oil can be reaped topically, applied directly to wounds, or even through burning; the smoke from the oil may help destroy airborne germs. Internal use will help keep the wounds from becoming infections, while external use will support the body's natural function in inhibiting tetanus.

Anticoagulant

As an anticoagulant, helichrysum essential oil combats blood clotting, which can protect against potential wellness issues like ischemic stroke, pulmonary embolism, deep vein thrombosis, and myocardial infarction.

Anti-inflammatory

External or internal inflammation can be reduced through the use of helichrysum essential oil. For instance, if you or your patient has swollen fingers from arthritis or a swollen knee from a sport's injury, oral application of helichrysum essential oil may decrease irritation or redness, while also soothing the pain that accompanies inflammation.

Antibacterial

Helichrysum's antibacterial properties make it a powerful protectant against diseases produced by bacteria, such as oral, digestive and urinary tract bacterial infection. What's great is that, unlike some prescription drugs, helichrysum has no ill effects on body wellness or on the healthy natural flora that exists within the stomach and intestines. Click here to read a study on the oil's antibacterial properties.

Antifungal

While bacteria and viruses are plenty evil, fungi commonly lead to the most deadly infections, whether external or internal. Your ears, throat and nose are the most likely to become infected by fungi, the infections of which can be both excruciating and unsightly. If left untreated, fungal infections can kill, as they may spread to the brain. Helichrysum essential oil protects against these infections and more and is particularly effective against skin infections. Click here to read a study on the oil's antifungal properties.

Antiviral

The antiviral protection that helichrysum essential oil grants will essentially empower the immune system, building up a tougher wall of security that most colds, measles or mumps are unlikely to scale. This immune stimulant will ensure that your body is better prepared to protect against deadly viral infections.

Antispasmodic

The antispasmodic properties of helichrysum essential oil make it beneficial to such wellness issues as chronic coughing and other respiratory conditions, along with surgical processes, such as colonoscopy and gastroscopy.

Anti-allergenic

Combining both the anti-inflammatory and antispasmodic properties culminates in an anti-allergenic effect against hyperactive allergies or reactions to external catalysts. As an antispasmodic, helichrysum calms the reaction and, as an anti-inflammatory, the allergy's severity is relieved and reduced. In the case of throat swelling, anaphylactic shock or other severe allergic reactions, this anti-allergenic effect is, quite literally, a life-saver.

Anti-catarrhal

Catarrhal inflammation occurs when the mucous membranes in the body's airways or cavity are inflamed. This can cause a lot of mucous and white blood cells building up in response to an infection. The symptom comes with coughs, the common cold, infections of the ear, adenoids, tonsils and sinus. The phlegm issue can potentially become chronic, so addressing it early on with an anti-catarrhal, like helichrysum, is a proactive measure to take towards recovery.

Astringent

For those who do not know what an astringent is, it's a chemical compound that shrinks body tissues, which means it can aid skin issues and irritations, everything from acne to insect bites. The astringent property of helichrysum essential oil benefits everything from skin to hair to gums to muscles to intestines. As an astringent, helichrysum is an anti-agent, combating muscle loss through the ability to strengthen. This astringent property also mean that diarrhea can be relieved through application of helichrysum essential oil, as well as wound and cut bleeding.

Nervine

As a nervine, helichrysum helps calm nervous convulsions and nervous conditions, like anxiety, hysteria, and vertigo.

Diuretic

If you're looking to lose water weight and reduce blood pressure, helichrysum essential oil is your agent. The oil stimulates urination, promoting not only the loss of water weight, but the loss of fats, uric acid, sodium, and other body toxins.

Expectorant

Throat or respiratory infections can be relieved through the use of helichrysum essential oil. Acting as an expectorant, helichrysum breaks up and helps destroy the phlegm and mucus buildup that accompanies sinuses or respiratory infections. Inflamed throat and lungs – and, thus, coughing – can also be alleviated through the application of this oil.

Mucolytic

A mucolytic is a substance that helps dissolve large amounts of mucus, supporting proper breathing by clearing up the respiratory pathways. Helichrysum essential oil can thereby serve those suffering from coughing.

Cicatrisant

Applied topically, helichrysum is effective when it comes to skin issues. The oil fades scars and other skin imperfections, such as acne, boils, stretch marks, and pox. It's also an incredible anti-agent, reducing the appearance of wrinkles and sun spots, tightening skin and providing an even tone. It does this by replacing old skin cells with new ones.

Hepatic

As a hepatic, helichrysum essential oil supports the liver by managing the bile discharge and promoting optimal liver function. The oil also helps to protect against liver infections.

Common Therapeutic Uses

Traditionally used to enhance the body's defenses against inflammatory issues, helichrysum essential oil remains a significant support for arthritis and allergies, protecting against inflammation, pain, and swelling. Helichrysum essential oil supports overall wellness, while detoxifying the body and providing particular fortification to liver and spleen function. Let's take a closer look at the common uses for this oil.

Detoxifying Agent

Helichrysum essential oil is an effective detoxifying agent. The oil's components eliminate oxidants that enter the body through such environmental inlets as the foods we eat, the products we use, the air we breathe, the water we wash with, and other like factors. Toxins can cause numerous physiological issues, including heart problems, lung or kidney diseases, or even cancer. What helichrysum does to eliminate free radicals is to draw the toxins out and transfer them into the urinary tract, where they can be safely removed from the body. Thus, through the oil's high antioxidant content and its ability to stimulate urination, helichrysum helps cleanse and detoxify the body's systems. Click here to read a study on the oil's antioxidant properties.

Skin Care

Helichrysum essential oil supports the body's defenses against acne, wrinkles, scars, dryness, sagging skin, and other skin issues. The oil's properties invigorate dull skin, while cleansing and eliminating excess oil. Whether using helichrysum essential oil to defy skin aging or to reduce adolescent skin issues, like pimples and acne, the antiseptic, astringent, cicatrisant, and anti-inflammatory properties are superb counter-defenders for skin issues. Helichrysum essential oil also supports cell wellness and promotes the regeneration of skin cells. Click here to read a study that evaluates the oil's effects on animal dermatitis.

Respiratory Issues

As an anti-inflammatory, expectorant, and mucolytic, helichrysum essential oil calms coughing by opening the airways. Bronchitis, congestion, asthma, sinusitis, cough, and other respiratory issues can be supported with helichrysum essential oil, as the oil promotes respiratory tract function by soothing the throat and clearing nasal passages.

Cardiovascular Wellness

Cardiovascular wellness can be maintained through the use of helichrysum essential oil. The oil's anticoagulant properties protect against blood clots that result from hemorrhaging, while the thickening of the blood reduces the risk of heart attack.

Digestion

As a digestive aid, helichrysum essential oil's collective properties stimulate digestive enzyme secretion which serves to support issues like stomach cramps and infections. As helichrysum is often used as a spice, akin to curry or rosemary, the digestive properties are coupled with an enrichment of culinary flavor.

Relieving Allergies

Bypass those allergy drugs with their laundry lists of side effects and, instead, seek out the all-natural therapeutic relief of helichrysum. The antispasmodic and anti-inflammatory properties can help soothe and relieve allergic reactions, making helichrysum an good oil to have on hand for those with hypersensitive skin or sinus allergies.

Safety Precautions & Common Applications

Safety

Certain adverse effects may evolve when using pure essential oils. Some essential oils should not be used when pregnant, for example, as they may cause miscarriage. Allergic reactions, too, may occur, especially when applied topically. Always administer an allergy test before committing fully to topical application. When used with other medications, essential oils may react negatively. If you are on any current prescription medications or have a chronic illness, such as high blood pressure, epilepsy or liver disease, then researching the effects of essential oils against your own personal medical history will eliminate any potentially problematic issues.

Helichrysum has been approved by the FDA for internal consumption and so can be used as a dietary supplement. Helichrysum is an anticoagulant, so if you're using it alongside blood thinners, their effects will be enhanced. If you are pregnant, always use at the discretion of your physician. If you have sensitive skin, dilute heavily and test before extensive use. Otherwise, apply neat or undiluted. You can apply topically, diffuse or use as a dietary supplement.

Blends

Oftentimes, essential oils are manufactured as blends of several pure oils. For instance, the Protective Blend(a mix of cinnamon, clove, rosemary, and eucalyptus). This blend can be used to boost the immune system to help support colds, viruses and flus. The downside to blends is that the more oils added to the mix, the higher the probability your patient may react negatively to the blend if he/she is prone to allergies. There is also the possibility of phototoxicity when working with blends, particularly if they include citrus oils. Be sure to read your labels before administering.

Regardless of these possible effects, essential oils are a viable option for supporting a number of conditions. Those looking to support or maintain their own personal wellness, or that of their families', should become educated on the uses of essential oils, their natural remedies and the methods of application. Only then can you begin building your kit of essential oils for everyday use and preparedness.

Chapter 2:
Recipes for Helichrysum
Essential Oil

In this chapter, we'll offer various recipes for helichrysum essential oil, both for pure helichrysum applications and blends. For pure applications, we've provided the appropriate dosage and method of administration to support specific ailments, from aneurysm to wound care. When it comes to blends, herbalists and aromatherapists often combine helichrysum essential oil with ylang ylang, sage, rose, lime, lavender, geranium, orange, neroli, and petitgrain essential oils. We'll offer some fantastic blending options in the second half of this chapter.

Pure Applications

Abscess Tooth

To relieve the pain of an abscess tooth, apply one drop of helichrysum essential oil topically to the affected area, either directly inside your mouth or on the general region outside of your mouth.

Agitation

Calm anger, nerves, or agitation by diffusing helichrysum essential oil throughout the home. You can also apply topically, using the oil neat or diluted in a 1:1 ratio with a carrier oil and massaging into the solar plexus, over the heart, or in a full-body massage.

Aneurysm

To protect against aneurysm, use neat or dilute helichrysum essential oil in a 1:1 ratio with a carrier oil and apply topically, massaging over the heart and into the reflex points of the feet on a daily basis. For added support, diffuse throughout the room.

Anxiety

To relieve anxiety, place one drop of helichrysum essential oil into your palm and rub your hands together. Place your hand over your nose and mouth and inhale. You can also diffuse throughout your home to alleviate tension and stress, or apply two drops neat or diluted in a 1:1 ratio over the area of the heart and the back of the neck.

Bleeding

If you need to stop up bleeding - from shaving nicks, for instance - apply a single drop of helichrysum essential oil to the affected area.

Bone Bruising or Pain

Accelerate the healing process when it comes to bone bruising or pain by using 1-2 drops of helichrysum essential oil either neat or diluted in a 1:1 ratio with a carrier oil; then apply topically over the affected area (do not massage).

Broken Blood Vessel

For broken blood vessels, use neat or dilute helichrysum essential oil in a 1:1 ratio with a carrier oil and apply topically to affected area (do not massage).

Bruising

Accelerate the healing process when it comes to bruising by using 1-2 drops of helichrysum essential oil either neat or diluted in a 1:1 ratio with a carrier oil; then apply topically over the affected area (do not massage).

Catarrh

Relieve catarrh inflammation by using neat or diluting 1-2 drops of helichrysum essential oil in a 1:1 ratio with a carrier oil; then apply topically over the chest and throat multiple times daily. You can also inhale directly from the bottle for added support.

Cholesterol Levels

Promote better cholesterol levels by using neat or diluting helichrysum essential oil in a 1:1 ratio with a carrier oil and massaging over the heart and into the reflex points of the feet.

Colitis

Inflammation of the colon can be alleviated by a topical application of helichrysum essential oil. Use neat or dilute in a 1:1 ratio with a carrier oil and massage the oil gently over the affected area and into the reflex points of the feet, multiple times daily.

Cramps

Alleviate menstrual, intestinal, abdominal, or muscle cramps by using neat or diluting helichrysum essential oil in a 1:1 ratio with a carrier oil and applying topically. Massage over the affected area for cramping muscles and, for stomach, intestinal, or menstrual cramps, into the lower abdomen, the back, and the reflex points of the feet.

Cuts

To accelerate skin repair, stave off infection, and soothe pain, apply a dab of helichrysum essential oil topically to the affected area.

Depression

Combat depression by placing a drop of helichrysum on your pillow or in your water or tea. You can also inhale directly, diffuse throughout the room, or dilute the oil in a 1:1 ratio with a carrier oil and apply topically, massaging into scalp, neck and shoulders.

Detox

To support the body's systems through detoxification, use neat or dilute helichrysum essential oil in a 1:1 ratio with a carrier oil and massage into the affected area toward the heart and into the relevant reflex points of the feet. You can also apply 1 drop to a glass of drinking water and take internally.

Earache

Relieve earaches or infections by diluting 1 drop of helichrysum oil to 3 drops of carrier oil and apply topically over and behind the ear, but not within the canal.

Gallbladder Infection

Support the body's natural defenses against gallbladder

infections by using neat or diluting helichrysum essential oil in a 1:1 ratio with a carrier oil; then apply topically, massaging the solution over the affected area and into the reflex points of the feet, up to three times daily.

Hematoma

To subdue hematoma, use neat or dilute helichrysum essential oil in a 1:1 ratio with a carrier oil and massage into the affected area multiple times daily.

Hemorrhaging

Protect against hemorrhaging by using neat or diluting helichrysum essential oil in a 1:1 ratio with a carrier oil; then apply topically, massaging the solution over the affected area and into the reflex points of the feet.

Herpes Simplex

Combat herpes simplex virus by using neat or diluting helichrysum essential oil in a 1:1 ratio with a carrier oil and applying topically to the affected area and into the soles of the feet every day.

Hernia

Hernias can be targeted with helichrysum essential oil. Use neat or dilute in a 1:1 ratio with a carrier oil and applying topically, massaging gently over the affected area twice daily.

Hopelessness

If you're feeling dejected or hopeless, inhale helichrysum essential oil deeply and directly when needed.

Joint Pain

Relieve joint pain and inflammation by using neat or diluting 1-2 drops of helichrysum essential oil in a 1:1 ratio with a carrier oil; then apply topically, massaging into affected area.

Ligament Pain or Injury

Alleviate ligament pain and injury by using neat or diluting 1-2 drops of helichrysum essential oil in a 1:1 ratio with a carrier oil; then apply topically, massaging into affected area.

Liver Support

Support liver function by using neat or diluting helichrysum essential oil in a 1:1 ratio with a carrier oil; then apply topically, massaging over the affected area and into the reflex points of the feet. You can also place a drop in your drinking water and take internally on a daily basis.

Lymphatic System Cleanse

To cleanse the lymphatic system, helichrysum essential oil can be applied topically without dilution (if your skin is not sensitive) to induce sweating. Move from the outer extremities toward the heart.

Heavy Metal Detox

To detoxify the body of heavy metals, use neat or combine helichrysum essential oil in a 1:1 ratio with a carrier oil and massage over the liver toward the heart and into the reflex points of the feet twice daily. You can also apply 1 drop to a glass of drinking water and take internally.

Muscle Aches

To relieve sore muscles, use neat or dilute helichrysum essential oil in a 1:1 ratio with a carrier oil and massage the solution into the affected area.

Nosebleed

Stop up a nosebleed by applying a drop topically above and beneath the nose as needed. You can also daily apply it in this way in advance in cases of chronic nosebleed issues.

Pain

General pain can be eased by using neat or diluting helichrysum essential oil in a 1:1 ratio with a carrier oil, then apply topically, massaging over the respective reflex points of the feet in relation to the area of bodily pain or directly into the affected area.

Pancreas Support

Helichrysum essential oil promotes pancreas function. Use neat or dilute in a 1:1 ratio with a carrier oil and apply topically over the pancreas or massage into the soles of the feet. You might also use it as a dietary supplement.

Perseverance

To stimulate perseverance, place a drop of helichrysum essential oil into your hands, rub your palms together, cup them over your nose, and breathe deeply in and out for several minutes. You can also diffuse throughout your home or apply topically, using either neat or in a 1:1 dilution ratio, and massaging into the solar plexus. Apply daily for the best results.

Phlebitis

For vein inflammation, apply helichrysum essential oil topically, either neat or diluted in a 1:1 ratio with a carrier oil, massaging over the affected area twice daily.

Psoriasis

Helichrysum essential oil can be used to support the body's natural defenses against psoriasis. Apply the oil either neat or diluted in a 1:1 ratio with a carrier oil directly to the affected area twice daily.

Scar Tissue

Eliminate the appearance of scar tissue. Apply the oil either neat or diluted in a 1:1 ratio with a carrier oil directly to the affected area on a daily basis.

Sciatica

To target sciatica, use neat or dilute helichrysum essential oil in a 1:1 ratio with a carrier oil and massage the solution into the hips, from the center to the sides.

Shock/Trauma

Relieve shock or trauma by diffusing or directly inhaling helichrysum essential oil. You can also pour a drop into your hands, rub your palms together, cup them over your nose, and breathe deeply in and out for several minutes.

Sinus Infection

You can combat sinus infections by diluting 1 to 2 drops of helichrysum essential oil in a 1:1 ratio with a carrier oil, then apply topically, massaging the oil over the sinuses and into the reflex points of the feet. You can also inhale directly, diffuse, or apply a hot compress to the sinuses, incorporating a couple drops of helichrysum.

Skin (Dry, Sensitive, Eczema, Fibroids, Dermatitis, etc)

Helichrysum essential oil can support all types of skin conditions. Use neat or dilute the oil in a 1:1 ratio with a carrier oil and apply topically to the affected area. You can also add a drop of helichrysum to your daily skin regimen.

Staph Infection

Support the body's natural defenses against staph infections by using neat or diluting helichrysum essential oil in a 1:1 ratio with a carrier oil and massaging into the soles of the feet up to three times daily. This will cause your body to absorb the oil faster. You can also take capsules orally or add a drop into each meal.

Strength

Promote strength within by placing a drop of helichrysum essential oil into your hands, rubbing your palms together, cupping them over your nose, and breathing deeply in and out for several minutes.

Stress

Combat stress by steaming two drops of helichrysum essential oil in a pan of water, remove the steaming pan from the stove, pour into a bowl, place a towel over your head and inhale. If you don't feel it's done its job the first time, you can reheat that same water and use it once more without adding more oil. You can also diffuse throughout the room or place a drop onto your shirt collar for portable stress relief.

Stroke

Enhance the body's defenses against stroke by diffusing helichrysum essential oil throughout the home or inhaling directly. You can also apply topically, using neat or diluted in a 1:1 ratio with a carrier oil, and massaging into the forehead and neck multiple times daily.

Swollen Eyes

Reduce swelling in the eyes by diluting helichrysum essential oil in a 1:1 ratio with a carrier oil, then apply topically in the eye area, avoiding contact with the eye.

Tendonitis

Alleviate tendonitis by using neat or diluting 1-2 drops of helichrysum essential oil in a 1:1 ratio with a carrier oil; then apply topically, massaging into affected area multiple times daily.

Tennis Elbow

Combat the pain and inflammation of tennis elbow by using neat or diluting helichrysum essential oil in a 1:1 ratio with a carrier oil, then apply topically, massaging the oil over the affected area. You might try contacting a masseuse who specializes in treatment of this issue.

Tinnitus

Relieve tinnitus by diluting 1 drop of helichrysum essential oil to 3 drops of carrier oil and apply topically over and behind the ear, but not within the canal.

Tissue Pain & Repair

Accelerate the healing process when it comes to tissue repair or pain by using 1-2 drops of helichrysum essential oil either neat or diluted in a 1:1 ratio with a carrier oil; then apply topically over the affected area (do not massage).

Varicose Veins

Reduce the appearance of varicose veins by diluting helichrysum essential oil in a 1:1 ratio with a carrier oil and applying topically in an upwards stroke towards the heart twice a day.

Vertigo

Combat vertigo and maintain balance by diffusing helichrysum essential oil throughout the home. You can also pour a drop into your hands, rub your palms together, cup them over your nose, and breathe deeply for thirty seconds. To apply topically, use neat or dilute helichrysum essential oil in a 1:1 ratio with a carrier oil and massage into the area around the ears, the back of the neck and into the reflex points of the feet.

Viral Infections

Strengthen your body's defenses against viral infections by using neat or diluting helichrysum essential oil in a 1:1 ratio with a carrier oil and massaging into the reflex points of the feet multiple times daily. You can also place a few drops in your bathwater or diffuse throughout the home.

Wounds

Support wound therapy by adding a few drops of helichrysum essential oil to into a spray bottle filled with distilled water. Spray over the wound. You may also apply a few drops to a spritz bath and soak wound for 10-15 minutes. Lastly, you can dilute helichrysum in a 1:1 ratio with a carrier oil and apply over the affected area.

Blends

Arthritic Massage Oil

Ingredients

- 2 drops Black Pepper Essential Oil

- 2 drops Ginger Essential Oil

- 3 drops Coriander Essential Oil

- 4 drops Helichrysum Essential Oil

- 5 drops Roman Chamomile Essential Oil

- 2 ounces Carrier Oil

Directions

To relieve arthritic pain, combine all ingredients in a small bowl, blending well. Apply topically, massaging the oil into the affected area. Use as needed.

Brain Stimulant

Ingredients

30 drops Balsam Fir Essential Oil

- 15 drops Sandalwood Essential Oil

- 15 drops Frankincense Essential Oil

- 8 drops Helichrysum Essential oil

- 3 drops Melissa Essential Oil

- 2 drops Peppermint Essential Oil

- 1 ounce Carrier Oil

Directions

To help stimulate the brain, combine all ingredients in a small glass bottle or container and blend well. When needed, apply 10-12 drops of the blend per ounce of carrier oil and massage into the temples, forehead, back of the neck, and into the reflex points of the feet.

Facial Salve

Ingredients

- 6 drops Frankincense Essential Oil

- 6 drops Helichrysum Essential Oil

- ½ ounce Rosehip Seed Oil

- ½ ounce Carrot Seed Oil

Directions

To fade the appearance of scars or protect against scarring, combine all ingredients in a small glass bowl or container, blending well. Apply topically to affected area.

Gum Inflammation

Ingredients

- 1 drop Helichrysum Essential Oil

- ½ tsp Witch Hazel

Directions

In a small jar or container, mix all ingredients until well combined. Relieve gum inflammation by dipping your toothbrush in the combination and dabbing the salve gently over the affected area.

Headaches

Ingredients

- 3 drops Helichrysum Essential Oil

- 8 drops Marjoram Essential Oil

- 10 drops Peppermint Essential Oil

- 10 drops Basil Essential Oil

- 2 ounces Carrier Oil

Directions

To relieve headache pain, combine all ingredients in a small glass bowl or container, blending well. Apply topically, massage into the temples, forehead, back of the neck, and into the reflex points of the feet.

Hemorrhoids

Ingredients

- 2 drops Clary Sage Essential Oil

- 2 drops Helichrysum Essential Oil

- 2 drops Geranium Essential Oil

- 2 drops Cypress Essential Oil

- 1 Tbsp Carrier Oil

Directions

To relieve hemorrhoids during pregnancy, combine all ingredients in a small bowl, blending well. Apply to the affected area then soak in a sitz bath for 10 minutes.

Hot Flashes

Ingredients

- 4 drops Helichrysum Essential Oil

- 6 drops Ylang Ylang Essential Oil

- 8 drops Hysop Essential Oil

- 10 drops Basil Essential Oil

- 10 drops Marjoram Essential Oil

- ½ ounce Carrier Oil

Directions

To relieve hot flashes, combine all ingredients in a small bowl or container, blending well. Apply topically to the affected area. Use as needed.

Muscle Ache & Pain

Ingredients

2 drops Helichrysum Essential Oil
2 drops Clary Sage Essential Oil
2 drops Lavender Essential Oil
2 Tbsps Carrier Oil

Directions

To relieve muscle aches and pain, combine all ingredients in a small bowl, blending well. Apply topically, massaging the oil into the affected area. Use as needed.

Pain Relief

Ingredients

- 1 drop Oregano Essential Oil

- 5 drops Peppermint Essential Oil

- 10 drops Helichrysum Essential Oil

- 30 drops Balsam Fir Essential Oil

- 3 ounces Carrier Oil

Directions

Relieve muscle or arthritic pain by combining all
ingredients in a small container. Blend well. Apply
topically, massaging into sore muscles or arthritic
wrists or knees whenever you're in need of pain relief.

Pregnancy & Delivery

Ingredients

2 drops Clary Sage Essential Oil
2 drops Fennel Essential Oil
2 drops Peppermint Essential Oil
4 drops Helichrysum Essential Oil
5 drops Ylang Ylang Essential Oil
2 tsps Carrier Oil

Directions

To promote comfort during labor and to ease delivery, combine all ingredients in a small bowl, blending well. Apply topically, massaging into the lower back, stomach, and ankles. *ONLY USE ONCE LABOR HAS BEGUN

Seasonal Allergy Blend

Ingredients

- 3 drops Eucalyptus Essential Oil

- 3 drops Rosemary Essential Oil

- 4 drops Geranium Essential Oil

- 4 drops Helichrysum Essential Oil

- 8 drops German Chamomile Essential Oil

Directions

To relieve or protect against seasonal allergies, place all ingredients in a bowl or jar and mix thoroughly to combine. Apply solution to your personal inhaler. Use as needed.

Scar Salve

Ingredients

- 2 drops Sandalwood Essential Oil

- 4 drops Lavender Essential Oil

- 6 drops Helichrysum Essential Oil

- 6 drops Myrrh Essential Oil

- 1 Tbsp Grapeseed Oil

Directions

To fade the appearance of scars or protect against scarring, combine all ingredients in a small glass bowl or container, blending well. Apply topically to affected area.

Scar Salve II

Ingredients

- 4 drops Patchouli Essential Oil

- 5 drops Myrrh Essential Oil

- 6 drops Lavender Essential Oil

- 8 drops Lemongrass Essential Oil

- 10 drops Helichrysum Essential Oil

- 1 ounce Carrier Oil

Directions

To fade the appearance of scars or protect against scarring, combine all ingredients in a small glass bowl or container, blending well. Apply topically to affected area.

Stretch Mark Salve

Ingredients

- 4 drops Lavender Essential Oil
- 4 drops Helichrysum Essential Oil
- 4 drops Frankincense Essential Oil
- 6 capsules Vitamin E
- 1 ounce Coconut Oil

Directions

To help diminish the appearance of stretch marks, combine all oils and the liquid from the vitamin E capsules in a small glass container. Apply topically, massaging over the breasts, thighs, and abdomen twice a day, morning and night, during the second and third trimesters.

Sunscreen

Ingredients

- 7 drops Myrrh Essential Oil

- 7 drops Helichrysum Essential Oil

- 1 ounce Carrier Oil

Instructions

For an effective sunscreen, place all ingredients into a bottle and shake. Apply every two hours when you're exposed to the sun.

Sunscreen II

Ingredients

- 12 drops Helichrysum Essential Oil

- ½ cup Olive Oil

- ¼ cup Fractionated Coconut Oil

- 1 tsp Vitamin E

- 2 Tbsps Zinc Oxide

- 2 Tbsps Shea Butter

- ¼ cup Beeswax

Instructions

For an effective sunscreen, place all ingredients into a bottle or glass jar and blend well. Apply every two hours when you're exposed to the sun.

Tennis Elbow

Ingredients

- 2 drops Helichrysum Essential Oil
- 2 drops Lemongrass Essential Oil
- 2 drops Peppermint Essential Oil
- 2 drops Marjoram Essential Oil
- 1 Tbsp Carrier Oil

Directions

To alleviate tennis elbow, combine all ingredients in a small bowl or container, blending well. Apply topically to the area of concern, massaging until completely evaporated. Then apply an ice compress to the elbow for 2-5 minutes.

Varicose Veins

Ingredients

- 1 drop Cypress Essential Oil

- 1 drop Helichrysum Essential Oil

- 1 drop Wintergreen Essential Oil

- 3-4 drops Basil Essential Oil

- 2 Tsp Carrier Oil

Directions

To reduce the appearance of varicose veins, combine all ingredients in a small bowl, blending well. Apply to the affected area, massaging gently toward the heart.

Wound Healing

Ingredients

- 5 drops Helichrysum Essential Oil

- 10 drops Melaleuca Essential Oil

- 10 drops Frankincense Essential Oil

- 10 drops Lavender Essential Oil

- Witch Hazel

Directions

To promote wound healing for small cuts or sores, combine all ingredients in a 10mL roll-on bottle and top off with witch hazel, shaking well. Apply to the affected area up to three times a day or as needed.

Chapter 3:
Helichrysum Essential Oil Studies

Many studies have been done on essential oils to uncover and prove their therapeutic qualities. In the case of helichrysum essential oil, many of the properties attributed to the oil (noted in this book and elsewhere) are quite often validated through research from accredited universities and published by reputable scientific journals. In this chapter, we'll discuss a small portion of these studies. It's important to note that our knowledge of essential oils is constantly evolving. Keep up with any recent research, as it may turn up even further valuable uses for these miracle oils.

Study 1 – Antioxidant Properties

In this study available on PubMed, the antioxidant activities of helichrysum essential oil were examined, with the following results: "The chemical composition and antioxidant properties of the essential oil and EtOH extract of immortelle (Helichrysum italicum (Roth) G.Don subsp. italicum, Asteraceae) collected in Montenegro were evaluated…The results of the statistical analyses implied the occurrence of at least four different main and three sub chemotypes of essential oils. Considering the antioxidant properties, the EtOH extract of immortelle exhibited similar potential as propyl gallate and quercetin."

The sole purpose of this study was to analyze the antioxidant properties of helichrysum essential oil. Antioxidants protect against free radicals and repair their damage. Although our bodies produce their own antioxidants, these often become damaged as we age, so introducing natural substances that are high in antioxidants into our bodies allows these nutrients and enzymes to assist in chemical reactions which destroy the oxidants or free radicals. The study compared the essential oil extract's antioxidant properties to that of propyl gallate, which has been an antioxidant additive in the food industry to prevent oxidation for products containing fats and oils since 1948. The study demonstrated that helichrysum essential oil and the essential oil extract tested are moderate antioxidants, with the potential to prevent food from oxidation or to detox the body of free radicals that lead to disease.

Reference
http://www.ncbi.nlm.nih.gov/pubmed/25766915]

Study 2 – Anticancer Properties

In this study published in the Journal of Oleo Science, the anticancer effects of helichrysum essential oil were examined, with the following results: "Helichrysum microphyllum Cambess. subsp. tyrrhenicum Bacch., Brullo e Giusso (Asteraceae), previously known as Helichrysum italicum ssp. microphyllum (Willd.) Nyman, is one of the many endemic species growing in Sardinia, Corsica and Balearic Islands. In the present work the composition of the essential oil...was investigated...The oil was tested for cytotoxicity on three human tumor cell lines (MDA-MB 231, HCT116 and A375) by MTT assay showing a strong inhibitory activity on human malignant melanoma cells A375 (IC50 of 16 μg/ml). In addition the oil was assessed for antioxidant activity by DPPH and ABTS assay."

This study aimed to assess the cytotoxic and antioxidant properties of helichrysum essential oil against human cancer cells. Helichrysum was found to have significant inhibitory activity on melanoma cells. Melanoma is a brand of skin cancer that develops from the pigment-containing skin cells, called melanocytes. Due to UV ray exposure, melanoma is a common issue for Caucasians who live in sunny climates, whose UV rays adversely affect these melanocytes. If the tumor hasn't spread and is small, melanoma can be cured when found early and removed. If it is advanced, melanoma can be deadly and causes about 75% of skin cancer deaths, with 55,000 global deaths in 2012, alone. These results indicate that helichrysum essential oil may potentially be used to support the body's defenses against melanoma.

Reference
http://www.ncbi.nlm.nih.gov/pubmed/25492232]https://www.jstage.jst.go.jp/article/jos/64/1/64_ess14171/_pdf]

Study 3 – Fatigue/Burnout

In this study published by the Journal of Alternative & Complementary Medicine, the effects of helichrysum essential oil on fatigue were examined, with the following results: "The objective of this pilot study was to determine the effectiveness of a mixture of essential oils (peppermint, basil, and helichrysum) on mental exhaustion, or moderate burnout (ME/MB) using a personal inhaler…While both groups had a reduction in perception of ME/MB, the aromatherapy group had a much greater reduction…The results suggest that inhaling essential oils may reduce the perceived level of mental fatigue/burnout. Further research is warranted."

The study evaluated a blend of essential oils, including helichrysum essential oil, in regards to its effects on burnout. Over a three-week period, data was collected from a control group and an experimental group. The control received a placebo (rose water), while the experimental received the blend. Participants used the solution they'd been provided with in an inhaler at home and work. The participants were then asked to rate their feelings of burnout on a scale.

The essential oil group had significantly larger reduction in perceived stress levels, mental fatigue and burnout. These results indicate that the essential oil blend tested can, in fact, influence the perception of stress levels and reduce feelings of fatigue and burnout.

Reference
http://www.ncbi.nlm.nih.gov/pubmed/23140115]

Study 4 – Antimicrobial Properties

In this study published in Antimicrobial Agents and Chemotherapy, the antimicrobial activities of helichrysum essential oil were examined, with the following results: "The essential oil of Helichrysum italicum significantly reduces the multidrug resistance of Enterobacter aerogenes, Escherichia coli, Pseudomonas aeruginosa, and Acinetobacter baumannii."

In this study, helichrysum, as well as some of its individual chemical components, were tested against Enterobacter aerogenes, Escherichia coli, Pseudomonas aeruginosa, and Acinetobacter baumannii. Enterobacter aerogenes is a Gram-negative bacterium which is found in the normal gastrointestinal tract and does not often develop into disease in those who are healthy. However, the bacterium can result in infections, particularly from certain antibiotic treatments, surgical procedures, or venous catheter insertions. These resulting opportunistic infections, although initially susceptible to antibiotics, can become rapidly resistant, which requires a switch in antibiotics in order to prevent the sepsis from getting worse.

Escherichia coli is a Gram-positive bacterium, which can cause serious food poisoning.

Pseudomonas aeruginosa is a common bacterium found in water, soil, skin flora, and in man-made environments. The bacterium thrive on moist surfaces, and so can threaten the hospital environment by finding a home on medical equipment, like catheters, which may result in cross-infection. It is, for instance, the bacterium which causes hot-tub rash. P. aeruginosa also attacks immunocompromised patients, infecting the urinary tract, airway, wounds, burns, and resulting in blood infections.

Acinetobacter baumannii is a Gram-negative bacterium, which can become an opportunistic pathogen, especially in hospital environments, infecting those with compromised immune systems. A. baumannii is highly antibiotic-resistant, putting it in the category of an ESKAPE pathogen (ESKAPE includes the following bacteria: Enterococcus faecalis, Staphylococcus aureus, Klebsiella pneumoniae, Acinetobacter baumannii, Pseudomonas aeruginosa, and Enterobacter species). Being that this bacterium seems to have risen to prominence during the Iraq War in military facilities, A. baumannii is colloquially called the 'Iraqibacter'. The bacteria is particularly relevant to those soldiers and veterans who serve in Afghanistan and Iraq, but a multidrug-resistant strain of the bacteria has found its way into civilian hospitals, partially due to the transfer of infected soldiers to these facilities.

This study found that helichrysum essential oil significantly reduced the multi-drug resistance of these bacteria. The chemical component, geraniol, in particular showed increased efficacy of beta-lactams, quinolones, and chloramphenicol, which are the core constituents to several antibiotic groups.

Reference:

http://www.ncbi.nlm.nih.gov/pubmed/19258278]

http://www.ncbi.nlm.nih.gov/pmc/articles/PMC2681508/pdf/0919-08.pdf]

Study 5 – Antifungal Activity

In this study available on PubMed, the antifungal effects of helichrysum essential oil were examined, with the following results: "Malassezia pachydermatis is a common cause of more widespread dermatitis in dogs (CMD). Recurrences are common, and this disorder can be very troubling for both dogs and for the pet owner...The phytotherapic treatment achieved a good clinical outcome, and no recurrence of skin disorders on day 180th was recorded. This herbal remedy appeared to be a safe tool for limiting recurrences of CMD."

The objective of this study was to evaluate the effects of a salve containing a number of essential oils on the yeast, Malassezia pachydermatis, a significant pathogen in veterinary medicine, causing otitis and seborrhoeic dermatitis in its host. Canines are affected by this yeast, and the symptoms of otitis include abnormal odor, excessive head-shaking and scratching, and a dark colored wax build-up in the ear canal, while the symptoms of seborrhoeic dermatitis include scaly lesions and dandruff.

The study tested twenty dogs affected by seborrheic dermatitis with a commercial essential oil blend composed of six essential oils, including helichrysum, peppermint, lavender, oregano, orange, and marjoram, as well as coconut oil and sweet almond oil. The subjects were split into a control group and an experimental group, ten dogs per group. Twice a day for a month, the control group was treated topically with conventional therapy (a ketoconazole and chlorhexidine combination), while the experimental group was treated with the essential oil blend. The results showed that the dermatitis of both groups was significantly improved, without adverse effects. A follow-up visit after 180 days revealed that there were no adverse changes in the dogs treated with the blend.

These results demonstrate helichrysum's derma-protective activity and, moreover, indicate that the essential oil could potentially be used in blends to support animal diseases caused by pathogenic yeasts.

Reference
http://www.ncbi.nlm.nih.gov/pubmed/24746728]

Study 6 – Insecticidal Properties

In this study available on PubMed, the insecticidal activities of helichrysum essential oil were examined, with the following results: "Mosquitoes in the larval stage are attractive targets for pesticides because mosquitoes breed in water, and thus, it is easy to deal with them in this habitat. The use of conventional pesticides in the water sources, however, introduces many risks to people and/or the environment. Natural pesticides, especially those derived from plants, are more promising in this aspect. Aromatic plants and their essential oils are very important sources of many compounds that are used in different respects. In this study, the oils of 41 plants were evaluated for their effects against third-instar larvae of Aedes aegypti, Anopheles stephensi and Culex quinquefasciatus…Thirteen oils from 41 plants (including helichrysum) induced 100% mortality after 24 h, or even after shorter periods."

Prevalent primarily in the tropics, dengue fever affects between 50 and 528 million people annually and is endemic in over 110 countries. The infection is transmitted via mosquitoes which carry the dengue virus, among them the Ae. aegypti species. The resulting symptoms of the viral disease include joint and muscle pain, fever, and skin rash which is akin to the measles. The disease can sometimes escalate into dengue hemorrhagic fever or dengue shock syndrome, each far more fatal than common dengue fever. There is no commercial vaccine for dengue fever, therefore eliminating the mosquitoes' habitats and reducing exposure to bites is the primary preventative measure. Treatment of dengue fever, as well, is supported primarily through rehydration with no pharmaceutical medication yet developed to target the virus directly (although medications are in development).

Culex quinquefasciatus and Anopheles stephensi are malaria-carrying mosquitoes, while the former is also known to transmit West Nile virus. West Nile virus was first discovered in Africa, but now affects all corners of the world, including the continental United States, with 286 deaths in 2012, alone. Symptoms of West Nile may include fever, fatigue, headaches, muscle aches, nausea, vomiting, rash, malaise, and anorexia. Most of the global malarial infections are in Africa, with over 247 million human infections to date, worldwide, 98% of which occur in Africa. Malarial symptoms include nausea, vomiting, fatigue, headache, chills, sweats, and fever.

According to this study, helichrysum essential oil shows promise in the terminating of the virus-carrying mosquito larvae. The oil demonstrated 100% mortality after 24 hours against Aedes aegypti, making it an effective potential mosquito control in areas where dengue fever, malaria, or West Nile are endemic.

Reference:http://www.ncbi.nlm.nih.gov/pubmed/1664238 6]

Chapter 4:
The Ins & Outs of Essential Oils

Where do essential oils come from?

Plants and plant species naturally produce essential oils for various reasons, one being to draw pollinator insects to them, another being to repel invading organisms (bacteria, animals). A number of chemical compounds compose each plant's essential oil, and the combination of these compounds is specific to each oil, which then instills in the oil its own unique properties. Essential oils can be harnessed from all sorts of plant components, including flowers, leaves, bark, fruit, roots, and resin. For instance, cinnamon oil is harnessed from bark, lemon oil from the peel, and lavender oil from lavender flowers. Certain plants can produce a few chemical variants of the same essential oil, which are acquired from different parts of the plant.

Some of these parts produce a large amount of oil, while others produce just a smidgen. The oil's quality and potency depends upon a number of factors, including the subspecies of the plant, its soil conditions, the time of year and even the time of day you harvest it.

How are essential oils extracted?

Essential oils can be extracted from plants through various methods, including pressing, distillation, solvent and maceration. Let's take a brief look at each:

Pressing Method

Commonly used with citrus fruit, the pressing method extracts the oil through a technique which involves pushing the fruit peels through a press. Oily fruits and plants are best suited for this technique. Orange oil, for example, is extracted from orange skins through the pressing method.

Distillation Method

This technique harkens back to the days of old-timey moonshiners, as the same sort of method used to create strong liquor can be used to extract essential oils. Using a still, boiled water and plant materials will create steam which is then cooled by coils and condensed into a combination of water and oil. This combination doesn't mix, so the oil can then be extracted from it.

Solvent Method

Through a multi-step process, certain plant and flower oils can be extracted using alcohol and other solvents, which extort the essential oil from the plant materials.

Maceration Method

When a "carrier" or fixed oil or lard is mixed with the plant material and set out in the sun, over a period of time, the carrier oil is infused with the plant's essence. Heat sources, other than the sun, are often used to speed the process. Throughout the process, more plant material is added to produce a more potent oil.

How do you use essential oils?

Although some studies about the effectiveness of essential oils are conducted by small companies or even individuals, a number of them are conducted by the food and cosmetic industries. In general, the pharmaceutical industry shows next to no interest in herbal medicine, primarily because there are few options to patent such products. Being as such, the product's lack of profitability results in a lack of research funding. Regardless, the historical uses of essential oils tell us what we need to know: these oils have been effectively administered for centuries. The therapeutic qualifications of essential oils can be plotted in the survival of the human race across cultures and generations.

Another reason that studies on essential oils have not resulted in much conclusive evidence as to their overall effectiveness is because definitive results are sometimes difficult to prove, as the quality of each batch of oil can vary for a number of reasons. One is that essential oils are impossible to standardize. As mentioned above, even the slightest variance in soil conditions and the time of harvesting – as well as innumerable other factors – will produce a different product quality and potency. In addition, essential oils are often obtained from various species of the same plant; Eucalyptus radiata and Eucalyptus globulus can both be used in the making of therapeutic-grade eucalyptus oil and, as a result, they may have slightly different properties and degrees of strength or effectiveness.

Just as there are a number of methods by which to extract essential oils, there are a number of methods to administer them therapeutically. The variety of chemical compounds in each essential oil means that their benefits and applications also vary across the board. Below are a few of these methods.

Topical Administration

Direct application of many essential oils works like a sponge, as skin sops up chemicals and other things (like sunlight, for instance). Topical application is best when you want to clear up an ailment on the skin's surface or in the underlying muscle tissue. When applying topically, you may either massage the oil into the skin or simply dab on the skin for therapeutic results. You might combine the essential oil with a carrier oil for topical use in order to dilute its potency. This is safer, as the oil is so concentrated. You may support your body's defenses against rash or muscle pain in this manner, but you should always test your patient for allergies before applying. Adverse effects are produced by natural chemicals as much as synthetic ones; poison ivy, for example.

To test for allergens, place a drop or two on your patient's inner forearm. If a rash develops within 12 to 24 hours, then the patient is allergic. In addition, phototoxicity – sun exposure resulting in an exacerbated burn – may be an issue when citrus oils are applied topically. So one must proceed with caution when applying essential oils using this method.

Inhalation Therapy

Commonly known as "aromatherapy", this essential oil application is effective for inner ailments, like sore throat or cold. In a steaming bowl of distilled or sterilized water, add a few drops of essential oil and, with a towel over your head, bend over the bowl and inhale. The towel captures the vapors, making the technique even more effective. Essential oils can also be placed in a diffuser or potpourri throughout a room to produce somewhat diluted therapeutic effects.

Ingestion

When using this method, proceed with caution. Direct ingestion of essential oils must be monitored and applied in small doses that are diluted in a tablespoon or more of any carrier oil – olive oil, for example. If you are unsure of dosage amounts, make a tea with the relevant herb instead. Although the effects of this diluted use may be weaker, this application is a better alternative than an overdose of essential oils.

What are the general benefits of using essential oils?

Replacement for Prescription Drugs

One practical benefit for using essential oils is, of course, their substitutive nature; they can replace Rx drugs, which is the ultimate reason to educate yourself on their administration and to begin stockpiling your essential oil supply. One of the potential threats of economic or social collapse is the lack of resources, and primarily the inability to procure prescription drugs. Being as such, finding suitable supplements should be a priority when preparing for the worst.

Their portability is also a major bonus when it comes to survival prepping. The fact that these ultra-concentrated oils take up little-to-no space makes toting them to your shelter all the simpler should the need arise. And, because essential oils are highly concentrated, the application used in most methods of administration requires only a drop or two of oil, which means that tiny bottle will be long-lasting.

Cost Effective Supplement

Though money may be the last thing on your mind when it comes to prepping for a survival situation (money may even be obsolete in the event of social collapse), it is worth noting that the expense of essential oils pales in comparison to prescription drugs. Essential oils are a cost effective supplement to prescription medicine.

No Expiration Date

Another benefit of essential oils is that they do not expire, neither do they have "proper storage" requirements. A number of medicines and medicinal products must be replaced every couple years, so this sets essential oils ahead of the pack when it comes to shelf life.

Versatility

Essential oils also offer great versatility. Apart from providing therapeutic benefits, essential oils can be repurposed for household and hygienic applications. For instance, if you're looking for something that might serve your dental hygiene needs in a time of crisis, the protective oil blend is your go-to essential oil. If you want to maintain your skin's tone and condition, frankincense and lavender will do the trick; the latter also serves as sunscreen, so you can inhibit sun damage as well.

When it comes to the house or shelter, you can use essential oils to deodorize, which will come in handy in a disaster scenario where things might start to smell fishy due to lack of proper utilities and care. For example, after the 2011 tsunami and the subsequent nuclear reactor meltdown in Japan, a nurse named Risa Nakahira used essential oils to deodorize and sanitize putrid public bathrooms in overpopulated evacuation facilities. As relief workers searched for survivors, often wading through debris and decay, Nakahira also deodorized their boots and masks using essential oils. The possibilities of these natural oils are endless.

They are also versatile when it comes to the range of patients they're capable of supporting. The wellness of everyone from your great grandfather to your infant baby can be fortified with the aid of essential oils in the appropriate dosage. They even come in handy when supporting the wellness of livestock or pets. From teething infants to dementia in the elderly, from teenagers with acne to dogs with urinary tract infections, essential oils can serve any patient with nearly any ailment.

Conclusion

Now that you know all about what helichrysum essential oil can do for you – where it originates, how it's extracted, its benefits and properties, and the different methods of administration – you can use it confidently to support the body's defenses against wellness issues and start to assemble a kit of essential oils for survival. Essential oils can be purchased online or at your local holistic treatment store.

The various benefits of essential oils and their properties are countless. To build your own kit, first focus on acquiring the essential oils which may bear more relevance to your wellness issues or the potential threats within your environment. When it comes to skin issues, for instance, helichrysum essential oil will be one of your more crucial oils, due to its dermal-protective properties.

Used as a supplement or as your go-to for detoxification, cardiovascular wellness, or respiratory issues, the application of helichrysum essential oil in medicine has survived for centuries and will survive centuries more. When it comes down to it, you don't need to rely on pharmaceuticals; essential oils, herbs, and plenty of other natural ingredients can be used to help support any number of wellness issues, whether ailment or injury.

Essential oils are essential to your survival in the case of viral outbreak, social collapse or natural disaster because, when the SHTF, your access to pharmaceuticals will likely either be limited or eliminated altogether. Supplements to our modern-day standard will equate survival when no other option exists. And when it comes to a life-or-death situation, you can't let your wellness decline, no matter the state of the world.

DISCLAIMER AND/OR LEGAL NOTICES: Every effort has been made to accurately represent this book and it's potential. Results vary with every individual, and your results may or may not be different from those depicted. No promises, guarantees or warranties, whether stated or implied, have been made that you will produce any specific result from this book. Your efforts are individual and unique, and may vary from those shown. Your success depends on your efforts, background and motivation.

The material in this publication is provided for educational and informational purposes only and is not intended as medical advice. The information contained in this book should not be used to diagnose or treat any illness, metabolic disorder, disease or health problem. Always consult your physician or healthcare provider before beginning any nutrition or exercise program. Use of the programs, advice, and information contained in this book is at the sole choice and risk of the reader.

Made in the USA
Middletown, DE
05 July 2018